Upgrade Your Mindset
And Finally Get in the Shape You Deserve

By Devin Arrigo

Upgrade Your Mindset: And Finally Get in the Shape You
Deserve

Published by Devin Arrigo | www.devinarrigo.com

DEDICATION

Mom, you taught me to dream big and never to shy away from a leap of faith. Thank you for pushing me to write this book—your words mean more than you could ever imagine.

CONTENTS

1 MY FITNESS JOURNEY

My journey is unique and has taught me a lot about what it takes to get in shape.

2 REQUIRED TOOLS TO GET IN SHAPE

The two essential tools you need to finally get in the shape you deserve.

3 GET YOUR MIND RIGHT

11 powerful mindset attributes to adopt before taking a step forward in your fitness journey.

4 YOUR CUSTOMIZED STRATEGY

The Stacking Strategy: How to create your personalized training plan to achieve any fitness goal.

5 FINAL THOUGHTS

How to jumpstart your fitness journey and stay driven along the way.

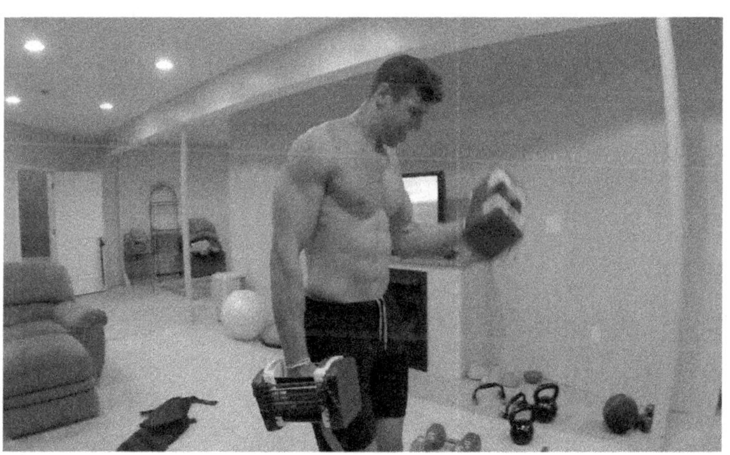

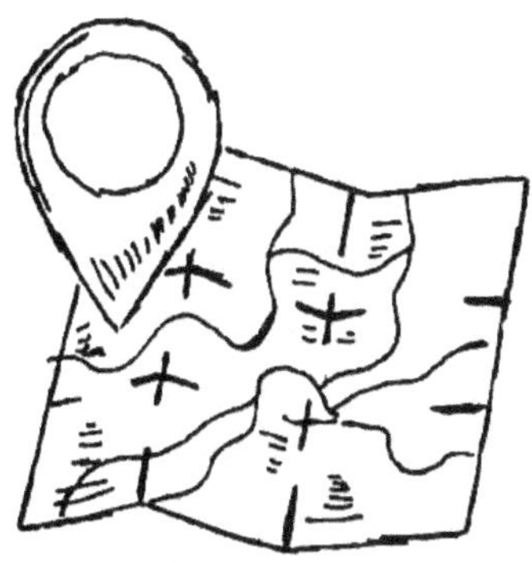

CHAPTER ONE

MY FITNESS JOURNEY

Fitness can be a lot of things.

To some, it's merely a means of staying healthy. To others, it's a hobby or a way to pass the time. And to a select few, it's a career.

To me, fitness is my best friend.

Like most kids, my relationship with fitness started in peewee sports. I can still remember the orange slices at halftime, my blue and yellow reversible jersey, and the thrill of scoring a goal in front of my family.

That thrill has stuck with me throughout the years. Since then, I've spent a *lot* of hours playing sports and exercising.

In high school, you could usually find me in the backyard practicing lacrosse. I spent so much time back there that the grass was ripped up, and my net was always torn and battered. But rain or shine, you could find me in the backyard, practicing my craft with my "best friend."

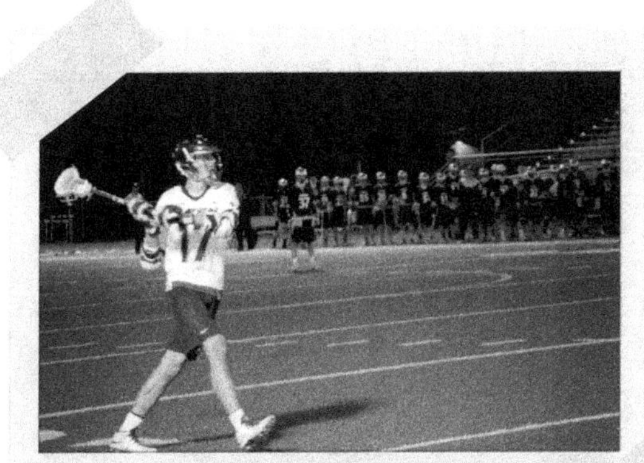

April 2014 - Senior year of high school.
Doing what I loved.

When I went to college, I lost the outlet I loved in high school and had to find a new one. Like many other twentysomethings, I stumbled into weightlifting and quickly discovered the lessons I picked up in my backyard applied perfectly to lifting weights. Soon I packed on 50 pounds of muscle and started teaching my friends how I did it.

Then, in 2018 I graduated from Penn State and started my first full-time job. As I balanced working and consistent weightlifting, I started to struggle with my shoulder mobility. After it escalated to being unable to raise my arm above shoulder-height, I saw a doctor who diagnosed me with nerve damage. There I was, once again, forced to find a new outlet and a new "best friend."

Because of my nerve injury, any activities involving upper-body movements were out of the question. My options were pretty limited, and having watched my Uncle run the Pittsburgh Marathon several times, I decided running would be my next outlet.

Over the following years, running became my new "best friend," just as practicing in the backyard was for me in high school. When things got hard, uncomfortable, or I was just having a crappy day, I relied on my training to help me get through it.

After a couple of years of consistent efforts, I've run a couple of short-distance races (5K's, 10K's), a handful of half marathons (13.1 miles), and two full marathons (26.2 miles).

Then, in 2020, I set my sights on a new goal: an IRONMAN triathlon. I'd always thought triathlon races were pretty badass and decided *that* would be my next goal.

Applying the same principles as before, I leaned on my new "best friend" and eventually completed an IRONMAN 70.3— a long-distance triathlon consisting of a 1.2-mile swim, a 56-mile bike, and a 13.1-mile run.

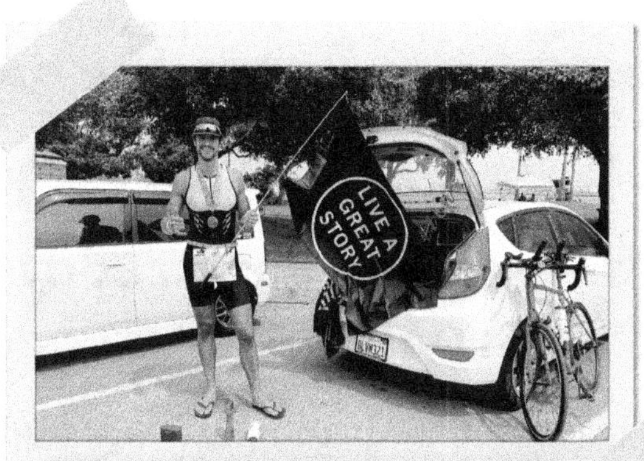

August 2020 - After my first IRONMAN 70.3 triathlon.

Developing Your Relationship with Health and Fitness

Like a best friend, fitness is always there for you. It's there to talk, bounce ideas off of, or just to lend an ear. It's honest, genuine, and always has your best interest in mind. It never lies or cheats. And what you put into it is what you get out.

Over the years, my relationship with fitness has evolved and grown. At first, I learned through team sports, playing lacrosse and basketball in middle and high school. Then in college, my passions shifted to weightlifting. And eventually, I found my way to endurance sports like marathon running and triathlon.

Each discipline has given me a unique understanding of how to succeed in fitness. Whether you want to get a six-pack, run a marathon, or play with your kids without getting winded—the principles are the same.

The Power of the Human Body is in What It Can Do

The human body is capable of more than you or I could ever imagine.

At a young age, I fell in love with discovering what my body was capable of. I loved the thrill of scoring a goal, making a great pass to a teammate, or getting more playing time without getting winded.

This love went deeper than just making a great play or the recognition that came with it. I was addicted to the feeling of pushing my body past what I thought it could do. I loved testing my physical limits.

I was addicted to finding the true potential of my body.

After nearly a decade of pushing my limits, I've learned that the key to accomplishing more in any area of life is learning to quiet the mind. Your body can handle more than you think. However, your mind will often try to convince you to quit way before your body's actual limits.

As former Navy SEAL and ultra-endurance athlete, David Goggins once said:

"Most human beings are only living at about 40% of their capability."—David Goggins

The human body is incredibly resilient, and if you can relax your mind enough to push through hard times, your body can handle it.

One of the most gratifying feelings on this planet is achieving something you didn't consider possible. It could be running a marathon, scoring a goal, doing more pushups than you've done before, or passing an exam you thought you failed.

When you push past your perceived limit, you learn what your body is truly capable of. This feeling is both empowering and enlightening. More importantly, it gives you the motivation to keep kicking down your perceived limits in all areas of your life.

I want to help you smash through your limits in life.

Health and fitness are gateways to achieving more in *every* area of your life. When you knock down one barrier, you gain confidence, momentum, and energy in every other area.

Learning what your body is truly capable of will positively impact every aspect of your life. An investment in your health is an investment in your *life*.

As the Greek philosopher Socrates once put it:

"It is a shame for a man to grow old without seeing the beauty and strength of which his body is capable."—Socrates

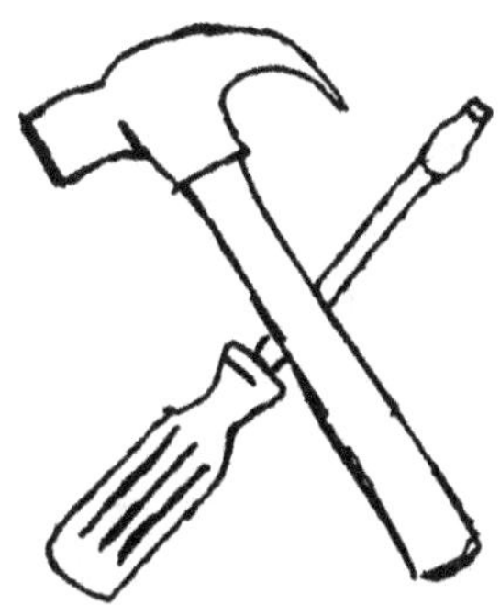

CHAPTER TWO

REQUIRED TOOLS TO GET IN SHAPE

Whether you want to run a 5K, hike Mt. Everest, stay healthy as you age, or play in the yard with your kids without getting winded, the principles are the same.

To get in better shape, you need two things:

1. The right **mindset**.
2. And the right **strategy**.

Without one, the other is irrelevant.

You could have the absolute best training strategy possible, but if your mindset isn't optimized, there's little chance of success. Or, you could have a championship mindset, but if your training plan is lackluster, you'll also fail.

In order to succeed, you need the right mindset *and* the right strategy. Together, they form the foundation upon which your health and fitness is built.

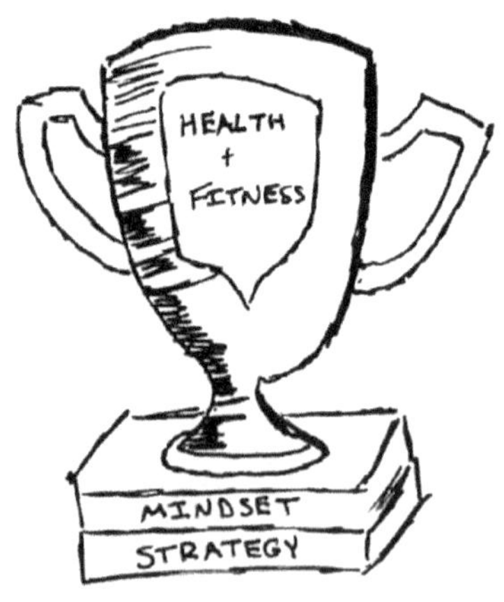

When I was training for my first marathon in 2018, I followed a very specific training plan. It detailed the exact mileage I had to run every day, the pace I needed to be running, and my rest days. It also slowly increased my weekly mileage to prepare me to run 26.2 miles at once.

I had the right strategy, but I also needed the right mindset. Some days I had to run at 6 am in the dark and cold, before I went to work. Some days I had to run 18 miles alone while my friends hung out. And most days, I ran when I *really* didn't feel like it.

Pushing through all these difficult times required the right mindset. Staying consistent required the right mindset. And finishing the marathon after suffering severe leg cramps at mile-23 required the right mindset.

After four months of training, I ran a 3:54 marathon, 6 minutes under my goal of 4 hours. I attribute my success to both my mindset *and* my training strategy. Without both, I would have never finished the race the way I did.

True success in health or fitness is the result of an ironclad mindset and a personalized training strategy.

In this book, I'll give you both.

After eight years of experimentation and practice, I've compiled the best tools and strategies I used to put on 50 pounds of muscle, run two marathons, and finish an IRONMAN 70.3 triathlon.

First, I'll show you how to get your mind right so you can succeed over the long term. Then, I'll explain *The Stacking Strategy*, a training method you can customize to achieve any health or fitness goal.

Let's get started.

23

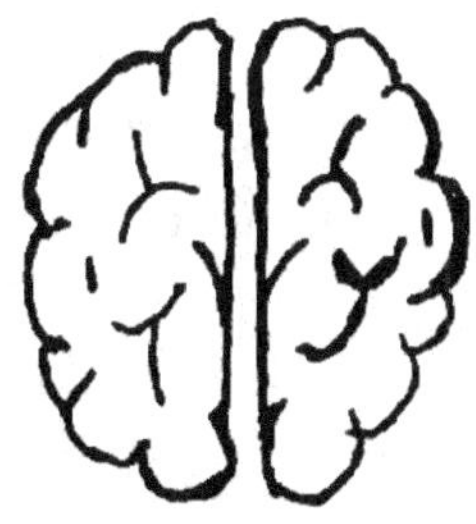

CHAPTER THREE

GET YOUR MIND RIGHT

You can't change your life without first changing your mindset. If you never change how you *think*, it'll be tough to change how you *act*. As a result, your life will continue to play on repeat.

Before implementing any training strategy, you first need to make sure your mind is in the right place. Without the right thought patterns, you won't have the drive or motivation to stick with a personalized training plan long enough to see results.

Ultimately, your mindset is driving the car, and your training plan is just along for the ride.

Here are the 11 mindset attributes you need to adopt before we can start talking about training strategies

1. Be 100% committed.

Before you step on the treadmill, lift one dumbbell, or even put on your shoes, be sure you're ready to actually commit.

It's not enough to say you want to get in better shape. You have to be willing to make a change to reap the incredible benefits of exercise.

If you really want to make a change in your life— whether it's getting healthier, feeling better, or even getting abs—you have to be willing to give something up. Continuing to live the way you've always lived will continue to provide the results you've always gotten.

There are no hacks, gimmicks, or tricks when it comes to getting in better shape. As Brian Mazza once said:

*"Nothing changes if
nothing changes." — Brian Mazza*

You can't expect your body to change if you don't take the time to change your lifestyle. To get healthier, you have to be willing to give something up. To make a change in your life.

What vices are you willing to let go of for a healthier body?

- It could be exercising 30 minutes a day, 4x per week.
- It could be swapping a takeout lunch for a salad you brought from home.
- It could be refusing to buy junk food at the store.

Whatever it is, no matter how big or small, to change your body, you first have to change your lifestyle.

2. Act first. Think later.

If you don't take the first step, you'll never get anywhere in life.

Incredible health *is* attainable. But, if all you do is *think* about getting in shape, I promise you, it will never happen. To get healthier, you have to stop thinking and start acting.

It doesn't matter where, in what direction, or how you start—to get results, you have to be willing to take the first step.

To get healthier, you have to start where you are. You have to do what you can, with what you're given.

- If you can't run 10 miles, run one instead.
- If you can't run a mile, fine, go for a walk around the neighborhood.
- If you can't walk, fine, try doing some bodyweight exercises at home.

Everyone is in a different place—different circumstances, different situations, different energies—but that doesn't mean you can't do *something*.

To get in better shape, you have to start somewhere. That could mean just taking the stairs at work, skipping out on dessert, or going for an evening walk with your spouse after dinner.

You don't have to pronounce "I'm going to get healthier!" then go run 30 miles. No—start where you are with what you can do.

The important part is that you start. Thinking is great, but if you never actually take action, you'll never see the results you desire.

3. Learn to workout even when you don't want to.

"I don't like working out" is one of the most common excuses I've heard. Whether it's fear of failure, embarrassment, or not knowing where to start, I understand where they're coming from.

Working out sucks 99% of the time. Even for me, it's not something I generally enjoy either. But with that said, it's something I do about 12–14 hours a week.

The reason is two-fold:

1. Exercise is good for you.
2. It also trains you for other things in life that you don't want to do.

Just because you don't like doing something doesn't mean you shouldn't do it.

- I don't like going to work some days, does that mean I shouldn't go?
- I don't like taking showers and going to the bathroom. Should I opt out of those?
- I don't like making food. Should I skip that as well?

There are always going to be things in life that we don't like to do. Often, it's the things we don't want to do that provide us with the most benefit of all. And working out is no different.

Treat your workout like a job. Or like a shower. Or just treat it like something you *have* to do regardless of what's going on in your life.

I don't know many people that go more than a day without showering. So why do we go weeks, sometimes even months, without working out?

Stop making excuses and just start doing it. "I don't like it" is not a good excuse.

Your health should be important to you. I don't care if you have to force yourself to do it, find an accountability partner, or make a pact with yourself —find a way to get your workouts in.

While you may not always like it, the return on your time will be incredible! In addition to the improved physique, you'll feel better, have more confidence, and find greater mental clarity, especially when other "don't want to's" arise in your life.

4. Don't compare your journey to others.

Comparison is hard-wired into our DNA.

According to the social comparison theory, it's one of the main ways we make sense of the world around us. 50+ years of psychological research shows that social comparisons form one of the cornerstones of social cognition.

What this means is that it's normal to compare ourselves to others. We do it every day to understand how we fit into the rest of the world.

However, with the addition of countless social media platforms, it's become nearly impossible *not* to compare ourselves to others. We're constantly bombarded with pictures of fit couples, rock-hard abs, and people living the good life.

Don't get me wrong—these posts can sometimes give us the information, motivation, and kick in the butt we need to get started. However, seeing someone that's ultra-successful can also have the opposite effect, only pushing us deeper into the path of least resistance and farther from our goal.

To get in better shape, we need to redesign our built-in comparison habit.

Instead of looking towards others, compare yourself to who you once were. Using other peoples' fitness as a benchmark is an ineffective way to get in better shape. Everyone is unique and has a different story. Everyone is starting from a different point in life. From a different perspective.

Take James Lawrence, for example. In the midst of completing 50 IRONMAN triathlons, in 50 consecutive days, through all 50 U.S. States, he proclaimed:

"Everyone's hard is different and unique to you, depending on where you are on your journey. Your hard could be a 1:59 marathon, or it could be getting up off the couch and going for a walk."
— James "The Iron Cowboy" Lawrence

Because everyone has a different starting point, comparing yourself to others is not helpful at the start of your fitness journey.

According to a recent study at Dartmouth University, "frequent social comparisons were associated with a range of destructive emotions and behaviors, including those directed at the self."

This means that comparing yourself to others could prevent you from taking the action required to get in better shape.

With a huge gap between where you are and where you want to be, this destructive emotion can take the form of self-pity, overwhelm, or even self-sabotage —ultimately resulting in you doing nothing.

Put down your phone. Stop comparing your journey to other peoples'. Start looking at your past self to track your progress.

5. Use motivation to stay consistent.

Former collegiate athlete and motivational speaker, Inky Johnson, once stated:

"Commitment is staying true to what you said you would do long after the mood that you said it in has left." — Inky Johnson

Motivation will come and go. While it's helpful to get started, we can't rely solely on it to propel us forward. All too often, motivation leads us down an unsustainable path of doing too much too soon.

Although our intentions are good, major overhaul changes are difficult to stick to and unsustainable in the long-run. **The most effective exercise plan is the one you'll actually stick to.**

Going from 0 to 100 in a single day is a sure-fire way to burn yourself out. You have to give your body time to adapt. You have to build a habit before you can build a chiseled chest or a rock-solid core.

If the goal is to get in better shape, the training method isn't as important so long as you can stick with it for a long time. **Consistency matters more than how much or what kind of training you're doing.**

Regardless of the goal, consistency above all else is the best strategy to get there.

So should you avoid motivation altogether?

Absolutely not. When the motivation strikes, take advantage of it and let it propel you forward. But keep in mind, the goal is consistency over the long-term. If you don't think you can sustain your current level of workouts, dial it back slightly.

One workout won't make or break you. Consistently working out over weeks, months, and years will.

Rome wasn't built in a day. And neither are the healthiest versions of ourselves. It takes time, consistency, and dedication. Find a training method you enjoy, stay consistent, and the results will come —I promise.

6. Train for something, don't work out.

Working out is *boring*.

Training for a marathon, a big ski trip with your college buddies, or to play with your kids in the yard —is exciting. Don't just workout. **Set a goal and then train to make it happen.**

It's easier to stay consistent when you're training for something meaningful. "Getting healthy" isn't motivating or exciting. Running a marathon to set an example for your kids is.

If you don't know where you're going, you won't know how to get there. Before you start exercising, set a goal for yourself. It could be to lose 10 pounds, run a 5K, or walk around the block every day.

Without a goal, you'll exercise aimlessly and end up nowhere. Thomas Carlyle summed it up perfectly when he said:

"A man without a goal is like a ship without a rudder." — Thomas Carlyle

7. Don't waste time thinking about your gear.

People who want to get in better shape talk frequently about getting healthier, losing weight, and starting to exercise more. However, more often than not, they get stuck *planning to get healthy* rather than executing it.

Let me explain.

Let's say Joe is super interested in running—which would be a great way for him to build healthier habits. Joe loves to browse the internet for the latest running shirts, sunglasses, water bottles, and hats instead of just going out for a run. He spends more time planning what he'll run in and where he'll run instead of running.

Like most people trying to get started, Joe spends more time planning and preparing than doing the actual activity that will make him healthier.

This type of mental hurdle isn't uncommon. Most people looking to get in better shape will generally experience 'analysis paralysis' — a state of overanalyzing or overthinking a situation so much that it causes them to become "paralyzed" in making a decision. This state of mind will limit your ability to take action instead of just doing it.

From runners to people aiming to look or feel better —there are millions of options or choices regarding shoes, clothing, watches, and equipment. It's tough to know what you actually need.

The best place to start is always with what you have. You don't need any fancy running shoes, clothes or technology. Just put on your favorite pair of shoes and do it.

The first time is *always* going to be uncomfortable. No amount of planning, purchasing, or prepping will equip you for that. There's no substitute for just doing it.

Heck, some people even run barefoot and enjoy themselves!

Don't get "paralyzed" searching for the latest shoes, shirts, or gadgets. Just go out and start exercising to build the habit. Eventually, the better gear may help. But don't let the lack of it be what stops you from getting started in the first place.

8. Don't wait for the perfect moment.

There may be a lot of reasons why today might not be the best time for you to start working out.

- *"Work is crazy right now."*
- *"The gyms are closed."*
- *"There's just too much family stuff going on."*

All of these may be valid and true. It's often difficult and uncomfortable timing. However, the people that stop waiting for the perfect moment are the ones that will ultimately succeed in their health.

Most people who are trying to get started are waiting for the perfect conditions. Waiting for a convenient time to get started. Waiting for the motivation to strike and push them forward.

This mentality happens pretty often. People who want to get in shape often wait for the conditions to be perfect, the stars to align, and the motivation to kick them in the butt and inspire them to action.

I get it, starting something new is difficult. Add in trying to change your habits and your body at the same time, and it feels near impossible. The perfect conditions would be ideal.

But, "perfect" is a myth. **The perfect time to get started isn't coming.** The conditions won't ever be ideal. "Perfect" is a fantasy—a hoax. The truth is, things are never going to be perfect or ideal when you're getting started.

The key is to embrace this lack of imperfection and *just get started.*

Putting off exercise while you wait for the perfect moment will only make things more difficult. Stop waiting for a convenient time and just start.

9. Don't be perfect, be consistent.

Consistency is the key to getting, and staying, in better shape.

One of the most popular misconceptions about getting healthier is thinking that you have to work out several hours a day. That's just not true.

I used to be a 240-pound weightlifter who couldn't run more than 1 mile. Now I'm 190 pounds and can run 10 miles with relative ease. **It didn't happen overnight, but rather through consistent, daily action.**

I consistently ran for roughly 30 minutes a day for a long time. And slowly but surely, my endurance increased, and I got better and better.

In all honesty, it doesn't take much more than 30 minutes a day to get in shape. However, it does require the *consistency* to workout 30 minutes a day *over a long period of time.*

Progress isn't made overnight. You won't get a six-pack in your sleep or train for a marathon in a week. Instead, progress is made through small, consistent changes over time.

Progress = Incremental Change (30 minutes/day)
X
Consistency (long period of time)

Rather than focusing on trying to be perfect—working out for X number of hours per day or working out seven days a week—focus on consistently exercising. Consistency is where real progress is made, not with the superficial idea of perfection.

10. Find something you enjoy.

Good health cannot be achieved in a single day.

It takes time, consistency, and a whole lot of discipline. If you don't enjoy your method of exercise, find a new one. Gardening, hiking, cleaning, walking the dog—there are countless creative ways to stay healthy and actually enjoy it.

Although sometimes you may have to force yourself to workout, you should start experimenting with different exercise methods to find something you enjoy. Doing something you hate for the sake of exercise is a great way to get burnt out.

If you don't enjoy what you're doing, you're less likely to stick with it long enough to see results.

11. Long-term vision.

Your health is a long-term game. You will not get a six-pack or get in peak condition overnight. It takes discipline, consistency, and time.

However, if you adopt a long-term vision, missing a workout or two, or eating a burger and fries, becomes *much* less significant.

For example, let's say you take a week off from exercise for vacation.

In the context of one month, you'll work out three of four weeks or 75% of the time.

Conversely, when viewed from the perspective of a full year, that same week-long vacation has you working out more than 98% of the time.

By having a long-term outlook, you're able to significantly reduce the impact of your time off. A long-term vision allows you to take more breaks with less negative impact on your health.

This is why Bruce Lee once said:

> *"Long-term consistency trumps short-term intensity."—Bruce Lee*

Short-term focus requires you to "hustle" and work as much as humanly possible. Long-term vision allows you to take your time and *slowly* build, making a sustainable, lasting change that will stick.

When you start your fitness journey, be ready to commit to the long-haul. Although short-term changes are important, long-term consistency is where you'll find the real results.

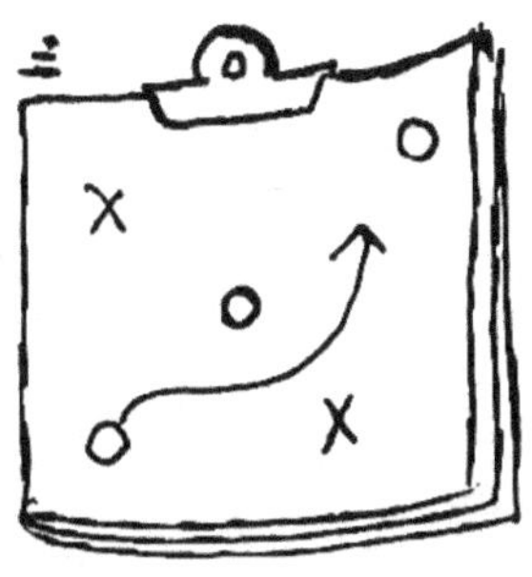

CHAPTER FOUR

YOUR CUSTOMIZED STRATEGY

I'm going to let you in on a little secret most people don't want to accept.

There is no "perfect" strategy or plan to get in shape.

What works for you might not work for your best friend. Or your Mom or Dad. Or your brother or sister. Your health is uniquely yours. It's a personal journey—one that I can help guide you on, but ultimately, one that you have to walk on your own.

The truth is, everyone is at a completely different point in their lives. Everyone has different priorities, time restrictions, health goals, training options, and fitness levels. Because of this, everyone requires a personalized training strategy that builds from *their* current fitness level.

Take John and Mike, for example.

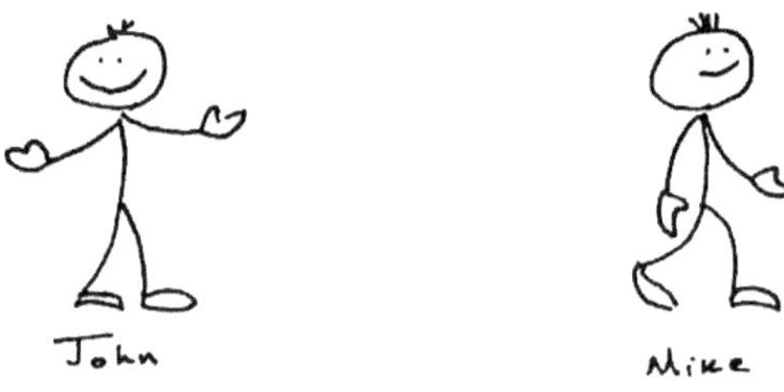

Let's say John is 30 pounds overweight and struggles to run a 5K. His best friend, Mike, has been running for five years and is currently training for a marathon.

Mike's training strategy won't be of any help to John because Mike has been consistently training for several years. What John needs is a strategy tailored specifically to *his* current fitness level. One that helps him lose 30 pounds first and then *slowly* builds his endurance over time.

Similarly, John's program won't help Mike progress towards his goal of running a marathon. Both John and Mike are at different points in their fitness journeys, have entirely different goals, and require personalized, unique training strategies to help them progress.

When it comes to your training strategy, there's no right or wrong, good or bad. Both John and Mike are working towards their goals, which is all that matters.

The key is to accept your current fitness level. From there, you can effectively build and develop. However, if you let your ego force you into thinking you can do more than you actually can, you won't progress the way you should.

Your "Norm" is the Key To Reaching Your Goals

A "norm" is the type or intensity of workout you are comfortable doing and requires little preparation or effort. It's something that you're used to doing at a specific frequency or volume.

A standard, if you will, that you're able to adhere to easily. A "norm" is something done so often that it requires little preparation or thought to complete.

Your "norm" is the key to developing the perfect personalized training strategy.

When I first started running, anything more than two or three miles was insane for me to think about. And honestly, it wasn't even something I considered possible. At the time, I was a 6'4", 240-pound weightlifter, so if I somehow was able to 'gut out' four miles, I was incredibly proud and slightly amazed.

In fact, at that point, I don't think I'd ever run more than a mile or two. Being a dedicated weightlifter, the extent of my "cardio" consisted of jogging to the gym and walking on the treadmill before starting my workout.

However, when a nerve injury abruptly ended my weightlifting career, I was quickly forced to find a new outlet. Having run cross-country for a year in high school, I chose running as my new way to stay in shape.

At the start of my journey, I was big, bulky, and *very* inefficient. I wasn't a runner but instead a weightlifter in search of a new outlet. Nonetheless, I was determined to get better and stuck with it long enough to see some results.

After weeks of persistent, consistent running, I slowly improved. From huffing and puffing on a half-mile run to running a full mile non-stop.

Eventually, I became pretty used to running two miles. It was a distance I felt comfortable with and was able to do pretty easily.

After a few more weeks of consistent running, two miles became relatively easy, required little preparation or warm-up, and was a workout I could complete in under 20 minutes. At that point, a two-mile run was my "norm."

After weeks and weeks of struggling with half a mile and then a mile, I eventually became comfortable running two miles non-stop.

Fast forward two years, countless hours, and even more consistent miles run, and I've now surpassed my previous "norm." In fact, I completely built a new one.

As of today, I'm able to comfortably, and with little preparation or thought, run 10 miles. For me to even think about that is still surreal. I used to be a 240-pound weightlifter who struggled to run anything over two miles. Now I'm 190 pounds and run 10 miles with relative ease.

That's the power of consistent, daily action. And more importantly, the power of using your "norm" to progress towards your fitness goals slowly.

I didn't create my new "norm" overnight. And it certainly wasn't easy. It took two years, a lot of hard work, and even more miles. But eventually, my body adapted, and running 10 miles started to feel like running two once did.

Rich Roll, an accomplished ultra-endurance athlete, summed up the concept of "norms" perfectly when he said:

"Every time we accomplish something we didn't think we could, that's like mental push-ups for the soul. You've then had that experience and your perception of your new normal shifts."— Rich Roll

The Stacking Strategy: Step-By-Step Method to Create A Personalized Plan

The concept of "norms" is incredibly powerful for getting in better shape. **More importantly, your "norm" is exactly how you'll create a personalized strategy specific to your goals.**

Because your "norm" is unique to you and your current fitness level, you can easily develop and grow as you improve your health. Once you identify your current "norm," then you'll slowly and consistently build toward your long-term goal.

The Stacking Strategy allows you to create a personalized health and fitness plan in four simple steps:

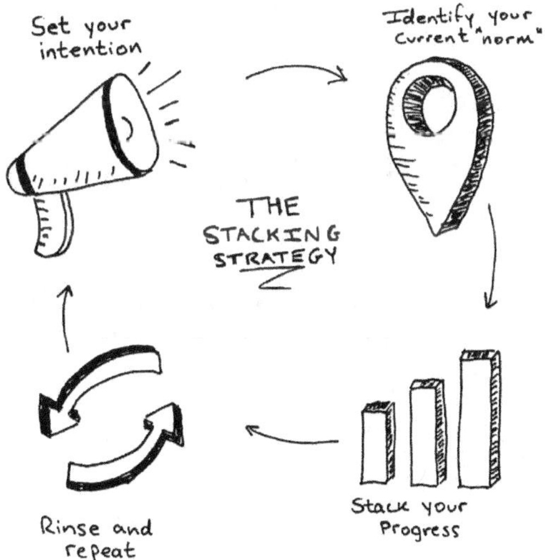

The Stacking Strategy starts by identifying your goals and your current fitness level. Then you'll slowly increase your working capacity to create a new "norm." Stacking one new "norm" on top of another, you'll progress sustainably and reach your goals in a way that will allow you to avoid burnout. Once you achieve the original goal, you'll make any necessary changes and then set a new destination.

Let's walk through the four steps of *The Stacking Strategy* in further detail.

Step 1: Set Your Intention: What's Your Goal?

Without a clear, defined goal, it's impossible to identify the action steps needed to get there. The first step in achieving any fitness goal is setting your intention. What is your ultimate goal when it comes to health and fitness? Where do you want to be in one year? What do you want to be able to do?

Do you want to run a marathon? Lose 15 pounds? Get a six-pack?

There's no right or wrong answer here. The beauty of this strategy is that it allows complete freedom and personalization.

The only restriction is that your goal must be quantifiable—whether it's time, distance, weight, or anything else. For this strategy to work, you need to track your current ability, progress over time, and then clearly identify when you've reached your goal.

Some good examples of goals could be:

- Run a 5K, 10K, half marathon, or marathon.
- Walk 30 minutes per day.
- Lose 30 pounds.
- Bench press 225 pounds.
- Do 25 pushups non-stop.
- Run an 8-minute mile.

Whatever your specific, quantifiable goal, write it down and stick it somewhere you'll see often. I have sticky notes on my bathroom mirror, in my closet, on my computer screen, and even in my desk drawer.

The more times you're reminded of your goal, the less likely you are to stray from the path when things get difficult or uncomfortable.

Step 2: Identify Your Current "Norm"

Next, identify your current fitness level ("norm") as it relates to the goal you set in step one. Take some time to audit your life and understand the frequency or volume of that activity that you're comfortable with.

The key here is to be *brutally* honest. Lying about where you're currently at will only hurt you. The more honest you are about your current fitness level, the better this strategy will work.

Maybe you can only do ten pushups, run one mile, or walk for 15 minutes. Whatever you're currently comfortable doing, that's your current "norm."

For example, if your goal is to lose 30 pounds, start by measuring your current weight. Then, identify all the health and fitness-related activities you currently do and are comfortable with. Maybe walking for 15 minutes is relatively easy. Or jogging a half-mile. Or maybe riding your bike for 30 minutes.

By identifying what you're currently comfortable with, you'll be able to easily create a new "norm" and track your progress as you move toward your ultimate goal.

Similar to step one, your current "norm" needs to be quantifiable. In order to see progress, you need to be able to compare where you *are* to where you once *were*. Be sure to identify your current "norm" in terms of numbers and figures, such as time, weight, or distance.

Step 3: Stack Your Progress

Next, take your current "norm" and make a small, incremental increase to it. Then, work at that increased frequency or volume until you become comfortable or proficient.

For example, let's say your goal is to run a 5K. If you're comfortable running one mile, three days a week, this would be your current "norm"—3 miles per week.

Next, slightly tweak your "norm" so one of the days, you run 1.25 miles instead of 1 mile. Then all you do is work at this "adjusted norm" (1-mile, two days a week + 1.25 miles, one day a week) until you're comfortable at that level.

The key is to avoid trying to do too much too soon. **The increase to your "norm" should be *incremental*. I recommend roughly 8-12% more than you're used to doing.** Any change greater than that makes it difficult for your body to easily adapt.

That said, you know your body better than I do. You can adjust the percentage accordingly—just be sure to be honest with yourself so that you're not pushing too hard too soon.

In the example above, going from 3 miles per week to 3.25 miles per week is an increase of 8.33%. The benefit of a small, incremental increase is two-fold:

1. It gives the body enough time to adjust to the increased effort and helps you avoid burnout.
2. It provides the brain time to adapt and accept that it can operate at an increased capacity.

It might take a week, a month, or maybe even six months. But eventually, if you stick with it, your body will get used to working at this slightly increased effort, and it'll feel as comfortable as your previous "norm" once did.

When this new, "adjusted norm" feels comfortable, you're ready to move onto step four. If your "adjusted norm" is still difficult, continue to work at it for a few more days, or weeks, until it feels comfortable and relatively easy.

Step 4: Review, Readjust, Rework

Once you've built your new and improved "norm," you can then continue to stack one upgraded "norm" on another. Because this strategy is customized specifically to you, the process has no clear ending point.

When you reach this "final step," there are two things that could happen:

- **Result 1: You achieve your original goal.**
  Congratulations! You worked hard and deserve to celebrate your accomplishment. When you're ready, go back to step one, set a new goal, and then work through the process again. The beauty of *The Stacking Strategy* is that it's repeatable and customizable.

- **Result 2: You're one step closer to the original goal.**
  Maybe you haven't reached your original goal quite yet, but you have made significant progress towards it. The next step would be to move back to step three and continue to stack your progress—building another new "norm."

  From your improved "norm," you'll then increase the working capacity 8-12% and continue to work at that level until it becomes comfortable. Rinse and repeat until you eventually reach your original goal from step one.

Examples of Crafting the Perfect Personalized Plan

The Stacking Strategy is simple, yet can sometimes be confusing based on the goals that it's being used to achieve. Let's step through a couple of real-life examples of *The Stacking Strategy* in action.

Example 1: Run a 5K:

- **Step 1: What's the goal?**
  Sammy has always wanted to run a 5K (3.1 miles) with her Dad on Thanksgiving morning. With a clear, quantifiable goal, Sammy sets her intention on training to run a 5K this upcoming Thanksgiving.

- **Step 2: Identify the current "norm."**
  Sammy runs very infrequently. Being honest with herself, Sammy admits that the most she could run at once is half a mile, and on average, she runs about three times per week (1.5 miles total per week). Sammy doesn't beat herself up over her current fitness level but instead is excited for the chance to improve it.

- **Step 3: Stack your progress.**
  Having identified her current "norm" as running 1.5 miles per week, or three half-mile runs, Sammy then calculates the goal for her new "norm." Staying in the range of an 8-12% increase, Sammy calculates her new "adjusted norm" as 1.65 miles per week (a 10% increase).

  For the next week or two, Sammy runs .55 miles, three times a week. She does this until her new "adjusted norm" feels comfortable and relatively painless.

- **Step 4: Review, readjust, rework.**
  After becoming comfortable with three runs per week (.55 miles each), Sammy then goes back to step three and calculates her new "norm" at 8-12% more than 1.65 miles per week. Sammy continues to do this, stacking "norms" until she can comfortably run a 5K.

Example 2: Get in "better shape":

- **Step 1: What's the goal?**
  James has been unhappy with his weight for a long time. After an honest conversation with himself, he finally decided it's time to make a change and get in better shape. Reading that his goal must be quantifiable and specific, James readjusts his intention to lose 30 pounds.

- **Step 2: Identify the current "norm."**
  Next, James audits his life to identify the current level of health and fitness activities that he's comfortable doing. Being honest with himself, James thinks he can comfortably walk 20 minutes, four times per week.

  Since his goal is to lose weight, he also understands diet is essential. James identifies that he eats fast food four times per week.

  James's current "norms" look like this:
    - Walk 20 minutes, four times per week (80 total minutes).
    - Eat a fast-food meal four times per week.

- **Step 3: Stack your progress.**
  James then takes time to calculate his new adjusted norms for both of his goals. Keeping to the incremental increase of 8-12%, James increases his walking goal from 80 minutes per week to 88 minutes. This means each walk will now be 22 minutes.

  Planning to *improve* by 8-12% with his fast-food goal, James recalibrates his "adjusted norm" as eating out three times per week. Although this reduction is a 25% change, James is confident he'll be able to stick with it because it's only one less meal per week.

  For the next couple of weeks, James walks 22 minutes, four times per week, and also limits his fast-food consumption to three times per week. He sticks to this new "adjusted norm" until it feels comfortable and relatively painless.

- **Step 4: Review, readjust, rework.**
  Once his new "adjusted norm" becomes comfortable and easy to stick to, James returns to step three and recalculates his "norms" for both goals. He slightly increases his walking time each week by 8-12% and also reduces the number of fast-food meals to twice per week.

James continues to repeat this process while monitoring his weight and reviewing his progress. Eventually, after several months of consistent effort, James reaches his ideal weight and celebrates losing 30 pounds.

Keep Your Ego in Check or It Will Sabotage Your Progress

The process of getting in better shape using *The Stacking Strategy* isn't complicated. *Set a goal, identify your current "norm," slightly increase your working capacity, then rinse and repeat.* However, it does require consistent effort and intentional action.

Using *The Stacking Strategy*, I went from struggling to run anything over two miles to completing two half marathons, two full marathons, and an IRONMAN 70.3 in nearly three years. It didn't happen overnight, but rather through consistent, daily action towards my goals.

I continually stacked small, incremental improvements to my "norm" year after year. The process wasn't always comfortable, and I wasn't always motivated, but the longer I stuck with it, the more progress I made.

All in all, it's really about staying true to where your fitness level is at *currently* and slowly increasing what you're comfortable doing. One of the biggest challenges I struggled with was letting go of my ego and accepting my current fitness level.

I often compared myself to people who were in better shape than I was. It was both discouraging and a waste of my time. I learned this lesson the hard way and don't want you to make the same mistake.

If all you can do right now is walk one mile. Good. Just keep walking one mile.

Eventually, one mile will feel like nothing, and then you can start walking two miles. Then, eventually, two miles will feel even more comfortable. Then maybe try running half a mile. After some consistent efforts, running half a mile will become easier.

See how it works?

It doesn't happen overnight, and it's certainly not easy, but with consistent action and perseverance, *The Stacking Strategy* will help you slowly build your new "norm," all the while becoming a better version of yourself.

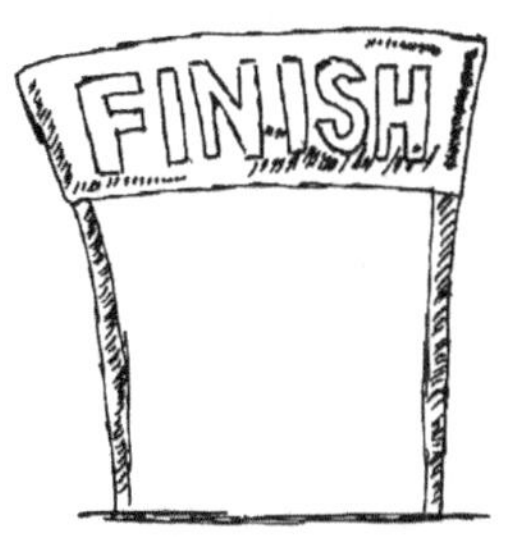

CHAPTER FIVE

FINAL THOUGHTS

The process of change starts with the realization that something isn't working. That something's broken. That something needs to change for the better, or you'll be faced with the worst.

My goal for this book is to help you identify any parts of your health and fitness routine that aren't working. And then to provide a simple, effective strategy to help you turn things around.

In my experience, most people understand the general guidelines to getting healthier.

Eat better. Exercise more. Treat your body like you love it.

It's no secret that the more you workout and the healthier you eat, the better you'll feel. The truth is, getting in better shape isn't all that complicated. It does, however, require a whole lot of discipline, hard work, and effort.

Your mindset is ultimately what determines your outcome. Consistency, discipline, and character are the things that will significantly impact your results.

If your goal is to get in better shape, first focus on adopting the championship mindset outlined in chapter three. Set a goal, fully commit, and don't be afraid to act. When the motivation is gone, workout anyways. Find a form of exercise you love, and above all else—be consistent, not perfect.

Once your mindset is ironclad, focus on slowly improving your "norm" using *The Stacking Strategy* **outlined in chapter four.** Set a specific, quantifiable goal, identify what you're currently comfortable doing, stack your progress by incrementally increasing your "norm," then rinse and repeat as your fitness goals change over time.

It won't happen overnight, and it certainly won't be easy. But as in life, nothing worth having comes easy. If you can stick with it, stay consistent, and keep a long-term mentality, you'll eventually be the person people come to for fitness advice.

At the end of the day, health is about forward-progress. As long as you're consistently taking steps in the right direction, you're on the right path.

If you hate working out, you've already missed the mark. Get creative, find a way to work out that you *do* enjoy, and stick with it for a long time. Good health cannot be achieved in a single day, week, or even month.

The truth is, your health is an infinite game.

There are no winners or losers. The trick is to consistently exercise—day after day, month after month, year after year.

The good thing about your health is that there's no right or wrong way to exercise—there's just the way that works for you.

If you love running, run often and consistently. If you love gardening, do it often and consistently. Or, if you love dance classes, dance often and consistently.

Find the thing you love to do, and do it often and consistently.

Working out for the sake of staying in shape is a dead-end. Life is short, don't waste it doing something you hate just to "stay healthy."

Find something you love, do it often, and stay consistent throughout the years—your body will thank you.

"Health is wealth."

About the Author

Devin Arrigo is a marathon runner, triathlete, online writer & self-development addict.

He is best known for his motivational style of storytelling and has accumulated more than 200,000 views on his writing to date.

In 2017, Devin was diagnosed with nerve damage that left him unable to raise his right arm above shoulder-height. No longer able to lift weights, he quickly jumped into endurance racing. Nearly four years later, Devin has completed a handful of half marathons, two full marathons, and an IRONMAN 70.3 triathlon.

Today, in addition to regularly writing articles online about health, fitness, and personal development, Devin works as a consultant, and also publishes a weekly newsletter sharing insight about both the mindset and strategies to get in better shape and stay that way.

You can subscribe here: www.devinarrigo.com

He currently lives in Los Angeles, but will forever be from Pittsburgh.